Health ZEN

Roditch Roditch

Contents

Introduction

Good health comes with discipline. "Freely chosen, discipline is absolute freedom." If you continue to eat junk food like you are still a child, your health will vanish by the time you are 40. You will be a regular visitor to doctors and hospitals, and this will be a hell of your own making—because it tasted so good.

Health used to be natural; now it's not. In the past, we had simple food, we exercised while we worked and played, and we certainly did not spend all of our time in front of a screen. With over 50% of all food contaminated with glyphosate (thanks to Monsanto) and other chemicals. With mobile phones, 4G, and soon 5G frying our brains and no protection from governments, we are now more vulnerable and sicker than we have ever been.

Most doctors know that disease comes from two places. The first is nutrition—the lack of a healthy, balanced diet. The second is the incredible amount of poisons on and in our food, in our household and beauty products, and in the air. This book is about my experience with health (and I personally should do much more to have extremely good health) and how we can all live to be 100 with a simple health plan.

I am encouraged to follow a healthy lifestyle after seeing what happens when you get sick and come under the care of a doctor. Some doctors are amazing, so you need to find amazing ones. But most doctors use questionable pharmaceuticals (no recommendations about diet or natural medicines). They do everything quickly so they can make more money, and they are driven by profits and prestige. What I have heard repeatedly is "Let's try..." This is their escape route. This reduces their chances of litigation and the truth being exposed, which is that they are not healers; they are pharmaceutical delivery boys and girls, and if the pill doesn't work, you are stuffed.

We are living in wonderful and woeful times; it depends on who you seek out for your health needs. There are a growing number of doctors adopting a more holistic approach and taking advantage of the extensive research and studies being done at the moment into herbs and nutritional supplements like CBD Oil.

In the negative, there is also GMO food, highly processed foods, super expensive health providers, microwave ovens, and glyphosate-saturated food that you and your family are consuming every day. There is also the pounding we get from 4G radio waves and, soon, 5G, which is 100 times worse than 4G, and our mobile phones, which is disastrous.

The money made by pharmaceutical companies is mind-boggling, and they have a lot of power over governments and doctors, which leads to corruption and poor advice from people we used to trust, like our family doctor and the government. Cancer is more prevalent now than it has ever been, but so are its cures. Thankfully, the internet is providing average people like you and me the information we need to take care of our own health, but not for much longer if Google and Facebook continue to censor natural healing like they are now. It is a revolution, and with CBD oil becoming easier to buy, I would say we, the people, are going to win. Everything is in your hands.

This small book will give you most of the information you need to have a healthy and happy life, but you have to decide whether you want to be in control of your life and health or put your fate in the hands of a doctor.

Simple steps to get started are organic food, pure water, sunlight, and fresh air. Exercise includes walking, sports like swimming and surfing, and running. Lots of vegetables, nuts, fruits, and seeds Some spiritual practices are like yoga, meditation, art, music, and church. A little sugar, alcohol, carbohydrates, and non-organic food a little TV, movies, computer games, and Facebook. I don't have a TV; they are the biggest time wasters. One thing I really love is reverse osmosis water with ozone by Singer, which is available at a dispenser near my house, and hydrogen water.

My father was born in the 1930s, and he was way, way ahead of his time. As a child, I grew up watching him read the health books that filled his bookcase. I can't remember him sharing his knowledge with the rest of the family; our diet seemed normal for the times. I do remember him telling me about people in the village he had cured with organic carrot juice, which was amazing. I recommend carrot juice to anyone who is not feeling well.

Take the healthy path and you will never look back. Have your turmeric and black pepper every day and ginger tea every other day. Drown yourself in pure Hydrogen Water and sunlight, take that walk to the beach and say no to anything you know will kill you sooner than later.

Most of the information in this book can be verified online through research and studies. We are now living in a good time because many natural cures and lifestyles have been verified by scientific research, which is published freely on the internet. There are enough herbs, supplements, and activities already verified by research to help you create your health protocols and change your health forever (without using anything that has not been fully researched), and there is lots more research coming.

"We don't have a soul, we are a soul and have a body," said George MacDonald.

""We are born healthy, we become sick." A quote from me. We are born healthy, and it is our natural state to stay healthy. Commercial interests bring us undone: packaged food, commercial home and beauty products, pollution, contaminated water, commercial farming for profit, doctors, hospitals, pharmaceutical companies, governments, politicians, supermarkets, pharmacies, nurses, schools, teachers, parents, seed producers like Monsanto, and chemical companies like Monsanto.

They are all what I call "merchants," people who want your money. I think you should always think about this when you are buying something: am I giving my hard-earned money, freely, to a merchant to support their interests of becoming rich and buying their next luxury home or car? Merchantism is a legal way to steal your money. Stay safe, stay happy, and avoid merchants at all costs.

To change you They are all what I call "merchants," people who want your money. I think you should always think about this when you are buying something: Am I giving my hard-earned money, freely, to a merchant to support their interests of becoming rich and buying their next luxury home or car? Merchantism is a legal way to steal your money. Stay safe, stay happy, and avoid merchants at all costs.

The Blue Zones

The Blue Zones are places documented by many people for their high percentage of centenarians. the Italian island of Sardinia. Okinawa is an island in Japan. Loma Linda, in California. Costa Rica's isolated Nicoya Peninsula and Ikaria, an isolated Greek island These places have many things in common: moderate exercise every day, small meat and dairy consumption, moderate wine consumption, lots of vegetables, especially dark green ones with plenty of calcium, and sweet potatoes. Fruit, nuts, and olive oil Two to three cups of black coffee a day are sufficient.

A general list of a Blue Zone lifestyle includes fava beans, red wine, coffee, empowered women, sunshine, gardening, no time urgency, likeability, turmeric, social engagement, legumes, constant moderate physical activity, a plant-based diet, no smoking, whole grains, cultural isolation, family, high soy consumption, little alcohol, faith, nuts, and healthy social circles. Low stress, low calorie intake, and a life purpose This is a simple, cheap, and easy way to live beyond 100 years. There is no better guide or reference than this for your good health and happiness.

CBD Oil

CBD oil is now mainstream in America and hopefully coming soon to the rest of the world. There is a lot of information on the internet about CBD oil, and I cannot recommend it highly enough for virtually all diseases, including cancer. This really is a revolution in health care and has been a long time coming.

CBD is one of 60 compounds derived from the cannabis plant. It is the major non-euphorigenic component of Cannabis sativa and belongs to a class of ingredients called cannabinoids. Our body has a system called the cannabinoid system, which needs cannabinoids to function. CBD is the most powerful form of cannabinoids and should be the very first thing you try if you are suffering from any degenerative diseases like cancer or Parkinson's. Stress, nausea, neurological disorders, diabetes, heart problems, leaky gut, and skin diseases all greatly benefit from CBD oil.

Other, but less powerful forms of Cannabinoids which are: essential oils of rosemary, black pepper, ylang-ylang, lavender, cinnamon, and cloves. Echinacea, truffles, cacao, helichrysum, omega-3 fats, kava, maca, copaiba, and holy basil.

The Five Elements

Earth, air, fire, water, and spirit These days, earth is something you find on a mountain or on a farm. Fire is keeping us warm inside and out, and the air is welcome as a summer breeze. Water is everywhere. Spirit is everything.

A simple way to look at your health is to consider these five elements of health as you make plans for the future. Have them all covered well. Earth is organic, natural, full of minerals like sulfur, and free of any chemicals. Air is fresh and freely flowing; it is not full of pollution like lead. Fire is the daily exercise that you love to do, like playing tennis, and it is a good digestion system with lots of healthy bacteria. Water is pure and natural, full of hydrogen, whether it comes from a natural spring or a reverse osmosis filter system; it is not from your fluoridated local water supply. Spirit is about peace of mind and joy and not about stress, fighting, or confusion.

Using these five elements guarantees you the freedom to be yourself and stand tall. Without them, you will be lost in the world of alcohol, sex, debt, and despair.

Water

Water is the most important medicine we have. It is still considered mysterious, and it does not follow normal scientific rules and analysis. Without water for a few days, we are dead, and with it, we live a tremendous life, full of energy and vitality. I love water—to drink it, swim in it, float on it, shower in it, watch it rain, watch it moving down rivers and crashing on the sand.

We are 60% water, so we are what we drink. Which one is better to be? Some chemical cocktail coming down the pipe or a pure, fresh mountain stream in the Rockies This is an easy answer for everyone, but we don't take the necessary action to create a stream because bottled water is so quick and easy. I recently started drinking reverse osmosis water with ozone, and I feel much better. I want to be able to drink bottles of this water every day and feel that it is totally safe and doing me good at the same time.

This water will flush out my kidneys and liver, cleanse my skin, and even flush out my digestion system instead of having a cleanout from my bottom, like an enema. Whether you are feeling very healthy or sick, it is so important to drink at least three bottles of reverse osmosis water a day with ozone or something better, like water from the Rocky Mountains.

Every single day, our mind tricks us so easily by saying, "I will do it tomorrow." This is your mind lying to you, as it does with so many things. If you are easily influenced by your tricky mind, then some meditation will help. These days I can hear it trying to trick me loud and clear, so normally I don't listen or act on it; sometimes I do, and always when I do, something bad happens.

Water is the number one medicine for all illnesses, either cure or prevention; do your best with it. Hydrogen water is very popular and is worth looking at. You can buy a hydrogen water machine or "Vital Reaction Molecular Hydrogen Tablets." There are also many things you can add to water like lemon juice, iodine (Lugol's), and colloidal silver. Wine, honey, and apple cider vinegar are also worth looking at.

Water is comforting, cleansing, and nurturing. If you are unwell, swimming in the ocean, having herbal baths, taking long hot showers, walking in the rain, and looking at the moon will reduce the tension created by unease, fear, and an overactive mind. helps you feel more connected and grounded.

Fire

The second most important medicine is the sun, or vitamin D. I have some old health books, and one of them has pictures of sick people in a pair of shorts sunbathing in a small hothouse. When I first saw it, I laughed to myself and thought, "Yeah, right." Now it's a different story for me and the millions who know we must have large amounts of vitamin D to stay healthy and strong. The sun is very important for our health, and we should not be afraid of skin cancer. The chances of becoming ill from a lack of vitamin D are far higher than getting skin cancer.

The fire of digestion is a major aspect of our health. Probiotics and prebiotics are essential. Every time you take antibiotics, your digestion system will be in trouble because the antibiotics kill both good and bad bacteria. Doctors never tell you this, so you can be sick for months with diarrhea, fatigue, and indigestion and not know why.

These are the best forms of probiotics you can take every day, whether you have taken antibiotics or not—they will increase your overall health: yoghurt, kefir, sauerkraut, tempeh, kimchi, miso, kombucha, pickles, traditional buttermilk, and natto. Gouda, cheddar, and cottage cheese can also be probiotic. All of these give you healthy bacteria in your gut and strengthen your immune system. Once you have lots of good, healthy bacteria, you need to feed them with prebiotics.

Prebiotics survive the digestion process and are different kinds of roughage: garlic, onions, bananas, oats, legumes, berries, asparagus, leeks, and Jerusalem artichokes. Probiotics and prebiotics are the easiest and cheapest way to maintain good health.

Another kind of fire is exercise. There are many studies that say exercise is the most important thing you can do for your health.

In the Blue Zones, everyone does some work every day, like tending their organic vegetable gardens. You will feel much better, stronger, and clearer if you exercise every day. It will increase the oxygen in your blood and make your muscles stronger, especially your heart. Fire is positive energy. We need fire to do anything: set our minds to a task, and fire will make it real. Many famous philosophers like Pablo Picasso have said life is action, and action is life.

Earth

Planet Earth is alive and is a system that needs to be in pristine condition for us to live here. We are part of the system—not separate from it nor superior to it. This requires every single person on this planet to take care of their own waste and their environment; if you can do more, then that is a huge bonus. If you continue to not care, then your children or your children's children will reap what you sow: pollution, poisonous food, 5G wireless, dirty water, extreme weather, and social unrest.

You have the power to do more; you have the responsibility to do more. Often our mind tells us: don't worry, the robots will fix it, scientists will discover a new way, I don't have time, it's not my responsibility. The truth is, if it's not your responsibility, then it's no one's responsibility.

The soil is the fruitful layer under our feet. made up of thousands of years of decay from rocks, trees, animals, and vegetable matter. It was natural, full of all the important minerals and elements that we need. Now it is a form of hydroponics; nothing in it is valuable. Every year, farmers fill the soil with fertilizers and mineral compounds, soak it in water and glyphosate, then sell it to you for large profits, paving the way to your future home in the hospital.

Your food should always be 100 percent organic or biodynamic. You can grow it yourself or buy it. It costs more, but in the long term, it is cheaper if you consider the doctor's bills and the long stay in hospitals you will have without it. Organic food is so healthy for you and your children that it tastes 500 percent better and lasts up to a week longer than mass-produced store food.

Organic farmers really care about your family's health and do their best to maintain the delicate balances of life in the soil, as do biodynamic farmers. The earth element is closely related to the merchants—the money grabbers. Land and land ownership have always been a way the rich control us—like the lords in England.

The rich and powerful have systematically taken land away from the American Red Indians, the Celts in Britain, the Australian Aboriginals, the New Zealand Maoris, and the Hawaiians. They fight over land rights at the South Pole and, soon, the Moon and Mars. The only way to counteract this is knowledge: learn how to be an organic gardener, make the most of small plots of private and public land, and grow buckets of yummy vegetables, herbs, and fruits—as always. IUTY: It's up to you; be strong and fight or give up. Take back the power of what you eat.

Air

We need air to live. Pure natural air, fresh from the mountain peaks, blowing down on all of us, living in the valleys. We need more than just life from the air; we also need good health. Our bodies thrive on oxygen, as they were meant to. Living in a natural environment is very important, maybe more now than ever. Pollution is extremely dangerous for your health.

Exercise increases the oxygen in your blood and improves your health on every level. Deep breathing with meditation is another great way to get extra oxygen. When we feel stressed, we often stop breathing (we don't know this). This is a vicious circle because a lack of oxygen will make us feel ungrounded and anxious.

One meditation I like is from the Alpha Mind System, which involves a sequence of slow inhaling, holding your breath, and exhaling two or three times. The technique is to breathe slowly in through your nose for 10 seconds, hold your breath for 10 seconds, and then breathe out slowly through a small hole in your mouth for 10 seconds. If you can, hold your breath for 10 seconds, and then repeat it one or two more times. If 10 seconds is too much, start with five seconds. So far in this book, everything you need to do to optimize your health is cheap or free: you just need to slowly change your and your loved ones' current lifestyles into ones that nurture and support a wonderfully healthy and joyful life.

Spirit

There is no life without spirit or soul. Spirit is the energy, and the soul is the identity. I would be lying if I said I had this sorted. I don't. My life is a constant search for meaning that brings peace and joy. Since I can remember, I have been a spiritual seeker outside the halls of religion. Some days I want to immerse myself in one idea, like Christianity, and other days I want to immerse myself in the truth of my own soul by developing my intuition. I believe in everything and nothing. To be honest, I don't understand why we worship a supreme being when we don't worship the creation this being created, which includes ourselves. My spirituality is about the earth and nature, about equality for all (rich people sharing profits with workers), about my own spirit, about being humble and helping others, and about being made in the image of God and feeling this deeply: "The devil is in your mind so clear your mind."

There is no health without joy, love, happiness, growth, sharing, belonging, and creating. This is by far the hardest but cheapest way to be healthy. You don't need to throw out your bibles and guides, but you do need to listen carefully to yourself and follow the guidance that springs forth naturally once the devil (in the form of negative thinking and fear) has exited your mind. Knowing the truth from deep in your heart clarifies all the wisdom and teachings over the centuries. There is no other way: be one with your soul, then, like a tree, grow up and toward the sun.

Leaves and seeds

In Thailand, leaves make up 20% of the diet in the cities and up to 40% in the country. In the West, we don't know what we can eat when it comes to herbs and leaves, which is a shame.

There are now books on the internet about wild foods and Thai foods. Yes, leaves are cheap and healthy and can often cure serious diseases. Papaya leaves are used as a malaria cure in Southeast Asia. Moringa leaves are a wonderful detox, and mango leaves are good for diabetes. Hemp leaves (blended in water) have many of the same benefits as CBD oil.

If you live in America, Europe, or Australia, you should study what leaves you can eat—the Aboriginals in Australia and the Red Indians in America already know many, if not most, of these. You will be pleasantly surprised at how much food is growing in your flower garden, in the local park, and in nearby forests.

There is an air of uncertainty about the future because of economic collapse, war, and environmental disasters. The Health Ranger on Natural News, Mike Adams, is a professional prepper. He supplies a lot of free information about preparation on his website, as well as incredible health information. He talks about foraging for food if the grid goes down or any of the above scenarios occur. You can learn a lot about living closely with nature from Mike Adams. You can also benefit financially and have better health by learning about all the leaves, flowers, seeds, and skins you can eat that you have been tossing into the trash all these years.

The seeds and skins of many fruits and vegetables are edible too, often being the healthiest part. Papaya seeds are good for parasites. Mango seeds are nutritious. Watermelon, pumpkin, sunflower, black sesame, flax, and chia are all very healthy.

If you search the internet for all your favorite fruits and add edible seeds, you will find a treasure trove of information about this topic. If you do a Google search using these words: "best book on wild edible food," a lot of good books come up.

Herbs

The revolution is happening right now. The scientific research into the benefits of herbs like turmeric and ginger is huge and getting bigger every day. There has never been a better time than now—internet, holistic doctors, and research—to take care of your own health: prevention and cure. The list of herbs confirmed by science is growing daily and verifying what herbalists have been saying and doing for centuries.

There are so many herbs that can cure our ailments. I am in awe of our planet and the universe and the idea behind their creation.

I cannot go into any depth about herbs as it is a topic that is fully covered on the internet, in books, and with many practitioners, especially Chinese ones. I suggest you type in your health problems with the words "herb" and "research," and you will find most of the information you need. The websites above, especially Natural News, publish new research findings every day, and it is the best place to start your journey.

In Thailand, there is little distinction between herbs and food. I think this is correct, and I have been a believer in the phrase "Food is your medicine" for a long time. Whether you are sick or just want to retain optimal health, I suggest you start your own encyclopedia of anything edible that has miraculous health benefits that could include: chili, turmeric, ginger, garlic, onion, astragalus, Andrographis, gotu kola, ashwagandha, ginseng, cinnamon, moringa, eucalyptus, honey, lemon, water, holy basil, sweet basil, carrot, cucumber, watercress, green tea, lemongrass, black pepper, pepper, peppermint, soursop, jack fruit, avocado, and there is more: dark chocolate, coconut oil, berberine, capers, mangosteen, beetroot, cayenne pepper, saffron, liquorice, milk thistle, grape seed oil, olive oil, aloe vera, lavender oil, Chinese knotweed, rooibos, bananas, flaxseed husks, frankincense, elderberry, cranberry, Indian gooseberry, mulberry leaf, thyme, kale, and All of these and more have been proven beneficial by research.

What you do is so important; balance your power with the power of doctors so you can be a winner with your health. Sad to say, I have no trust in doctors and hospitals because they are all about money. They do not optimize your treatment based on current research of all "effective treatments." They follow a narrow, pharmacy-based program because that is how they make their money, and they have all their pharmacy medical guides to use as a reference. When I was young, doctors did home visits. They really were more balanced in the past when it came to making money or healing a patient.

I recently read that a woman—who is not allergic to bee stings—went to an outpatient hospital in an American hospital just to be on the safe side after a bee sting and was charged $10,000 for a basic exam and treatment. The doctor billed her $7,000 and the hospital the rest. Affordable health care is impossible with this kind of corruption. I would suggest to any country they need to dismantle doctors' monopoly on health care and adopt three very simple ideas: up-train nurses so they can treat patients "independently of doctors" with normal and basic health problems (much cheaper for governments to fund), create a herbal treatment manual for nurses and doctors based on credible research, and create regulations about healthy and safe food, i.e., organic, use of poisons like glyphosate (supermarkets cannot sell any food with designated poisons in it) and pure drinking water.

I have been to the doctor once in 10 years. I trust my daily habits of taking herbs like ginger and turmeric, getting some sun, exercising, drinking pure water, and wanting to grow and learn more and more every day. You need to be strong, use this book as a starting point, and truly believe the new research that confirms natural healing works and works better than anything pharmaceutical companies come up with to make themselves rich and powerful. They are so powerful that they have a great deal of power over doctors and governments, yet they rarely ever heal us of any disease.

Food is your medicine

What you consume every day is the key to your health. It takes 30 days to change your habits, which is not a long time if you do change them and live to be 100 years old.

Organic fruit, vegetables, nuts, and seeds, along with pure water, air, and lots of sun, are where it all begins. Meat is a personal choice. In the Blue Zones, they eat a lot more vegetables and fruit than meat. Also, healthy oils like coconut, avocado, and olive are essential. New research about the cannabinoid system says we also need to consume cannabinoids like CBD oil. Daily exercise is essential, but it doesn't have to be excessive; you can work in your vegetable garden, go for a walk, or go swimming. Some forms of yoga and Tai Chi are other forms of soft exercise. Happiness is another important health requirement; stress is a killer. How can we be happy every day? Some options are meditation, doing what you were born to do, loving the partner you are with, reading, having good friends, living in a natural environment, developing your intuition, going to church or the temple, and paying cash for everything, including your car and house. Doing more things yourself, like building your own house, fixing your car, taking herbs and supplements for your health, finding the god within, and making an incredible fruit and vegetable garden.

There are two ways you can do this: the first is to rise above the financial limitations you face every day and become the best of the best at what you do and earn enough to pay for everything easily, and the second is to reduce your consumption to a sustainable level and revel in all the wonderful things you can do with next to nothing. I am in the second category most of the time.

You need to be thinking positively, throw out your TV, wake up early, like at 5 a.m., and go to bed at 9 p.m.

These days, when life is so complicated and technology rules, it's nearly impossible to believe that a simple organic carrot eaten three times a week can keep you strong and healthy. Back to basics and simplicity There is something quite devilish about technology, and I think it should be used in moderation. The building blocks of life do not include technology: health, love, family, growth, skill, wisdom, and humility do. If you ignore these, then technology will control your mind, which your mind loves, and you will be dependent on technology, and the merchants are creating more gadgets for your crazy mind to play with every day.

Simple is not easy. We can distract ourselves in a myriad of ways to avoid being simple. Simple ways to live include: cash, not debt; health, not sickness; wisdom, not ignorance; love, not hate; peace, not stress; growth, not stagnation; strength, not fear; and intuition, not mind. Food really can be our medicine; there are many books written on this subject, and as long as it is organic or biodynamic, there is nothing more empowering on this planet.

Trust

My father loved studying natural healing, back when it was unheard of. He had quite a library, which I loved looking at but never got to read. His interest in health was pretty amazing when I think about it, and it carried over to me. Neither of us ever went on to be practitioners, but our knowledge has helped many people for free. I still think about doing more, yet the average person is so untrusting and ignorant about herbs and supplements that the "sales pitch" needed to overcome this is so tiresome that I find it easier to disseminate information than cure.

I hope to impart trust from me to you in this book so you can take a giant leap into good health and happiness. I would love for everyone to have the best health care this planet can provide at an affordable price. The suffering that is imposed on us from without and from within is unnecessary and, in this day and age, redundant. I have not had a TV for 14 years, and it is the best thing I have ever done.

Try to avoid social networks and use the internet as your own personal library. Play a sport, help your neighbors, and your grandmother and grandfather—help anyone you can when you can. Investing in your wellbeing now is the best individual action you could ever take in your lifetime. There are a few obstacles: negative thinking (the devil in your mind) and lack of knowledge (now available everywhere). Take the power you are born with and become the master or mistress of your own destiny. Make a stand against the evil that permeates our world and become a shining, bright light of truth.

Trusting everyone who comes into your life in a pleasant way is important. Sometimes you will need to make a "leap of faith" when someone says they can help you with your health and suggest some herbs or supplements. Instead of conjuring resistance (which so many western speaking people do to express their superiority over others), have an open mind and think this is a blessing, and at least listen, take notes, look up these cures on the internet, and move on with them—do your best to get the advantage from other people's knowledge and love. I like the idea that God works through people. Talking about God, my understanding of him is limited, but I do know many religions and Buddhism believe in a God. I really like Carl Jung's understanding of the connections between people and unseen forces and energies, which he calls the collective. His ideas helped me realize that we are all connected and that we do work hard for each other on conscious and unconscious levels. This is what I call God: a collection of all spirits being one spirit and there being no separation. So, take the help gladly when it comes, accept that you are part of the collective, and one day you will do the same for others.

Goodies

All food is miraculous and delicious. My brother is turning 80 in a few months. He rides his racing bike 30 kilometers every other day. Last year, he came third in the world in a bicycle race in Austria. Recently, we had a long chat about health, and he said finding a balance in everything is a good start. He eats normal food (meat and three vegetables), exercises quite a bit, and stays away from most junk food.

When he was in his twenties, he was a champion tennis player, football player, squash player, and water skier. I said you are pretty amazing; you should write a book about how normal people can be champions, and he said he probably should.

He is a great example of how just a small shift in thinking can change your life. Change the program in your mind that says "I can't" to "I can." I love to do some exercise and enjoy the taste and benefits of healthier food over sugar, salt, and spices. A healthy life can still be fun; dark chocolate is incredibly good for you. Natural red wine is also very healthy, as are natural beer, natural grains, and sweets. Mediterranean food is so healthy: olive oil, olives, hummus, tahini, tabouli, babganoush, homemade pizza, seafood, wine, goat's cheese, kefir, cucumber, tomato, and yoghurt. There are so many delicious fruits, honey, beans, nuts, and seeds that the mind boggles. Food can really be your medicine. Medicine for your body, mind, and spirit Start adding more leaves to your food, like stuffed grape leaves, basil, chili, and lime. Vary your diet.

The Japanese have a philosophy about eating a large variety of foods to make sure they get all the vitamins and minerals they need every day. Asian fruits like jackfruit and custard apples are extremely healthy. Try to visit a different country every night when you have dinner.

There are so many incredible recipes for world food that it is easy to become a super chef. I was the main cook when my children were young. Men should cook as often as women. They can bring much-needed relief to a woman's busy schedule, as well as different menus and recipes, and have fun at the same time. In Southeast Asia, everyone loves cooking. It is a special time to wind down, relax, and be creative. Also in Southeast Asia, every suburb has a farmers' market. Everyone buys fresh food in the morning and evening; it is cheap and plentiful. Eat to live, and live to eat.

IUTY – It's up to you

Sounds hard, doesn't it? Being responsible for your life is called being "self-responsible." Using your free will in a positive way Working hard. taking care of yourself and your family. Making the world a better place Being part of the collective in a happy and joyful way Giving, knowing it will come back, increased.

Planting seeds and watching them grow Accepting your mistakes and learning from them Knowing your mind can deceive you on a minute-by-minute basis. Following the Christian and Buddhist 10 commandments: yes, they both have them. Being humble: all my ways are pleasant ways, all my paths are peace, and in quietness and confidence shall be my strength.

This is a topic I can honestly say I have trouble with because it's easier said than done. I can take comfort in knowing I can improve, and there are many good people and books explaining how to do it. It's up to me to stay on track and fight these invisible demons that keep appearing in my thoughts and eventually be free of them, like a samurai.

Comfort is a waste of time. There is plenty of time to be comfortable in heaven. I think we are here to create, change, make, fight, love, and live life to the full. If you like comfort—watching TV, eating too much junk food, playing games—then this is a waste of time on this earth, and I cannot see any reason for being alive. Get out of your chair and do all the things you think about and talk about doing; become a person of action. There is no chance in heaven to do much; it is full of angels and peace and tranquility, which sounds boring. Enjoy being a creator while you can. No fear: do it. Being healthy should be the first thing on your "creator's list." Create good health, strength, and power from what you eat and drink. IUTY—it's up to you. which basically means you and not another person or spiritual being.

I wish you all the best and sincerely hope that you, your friends, and your family have a long, healthy, and fruitful life, and this book is a good and strong stepping stone on your journey. Thank you for purchasing the book, and you are welcome to contact me on my website listed on the first page.

One last thing. The new outbreak of killer fungus Candida Auris that has no known cure maybe can be killed with ultraviolet light from the sun. I suggest if you contract this fungus lying in the sun for a few hours a day in your bathers while deep breathing will help.

Also, Covid-19. Some exceptional cures are hydrogen inhalation, zinc, Lugol's iodine drops, nebulized hydrogen peroxide (3%), and IV vitamin C.

Thank you for buying this small book.

roditch@protonmail.com

www.ingramcontent.com/pod-product-compliance
Lightning Source LLC
Chambersburg PA
CBHW051407280526
45784CB00007B/3130